QUINT … T SERIES

Oral Implantology Surgical Procedures

CHECKLIST

Louie Al-Faraje, DDS

Quintessence Publishing Co, Inc
Chicago, Berlin, Tokyo, London, Paris, Milan, Barcelona, Istanbul, Moscow, New Delhi, Prague, São Paulo, Seoul, Singapore and Warsaw

WATERPROOF AND WASHABLE
Write on the pages with a ballpoint pen only. Do not use marker. Use an alcohol wipe to remove information and reuse.

Library of Congress Control Number: 2012950978

5 4 3 2 1

quintessence books

Quintessence Publishing Co Inc
4350 Chandler Drive
Hanover Park, IL 60133
www.quintpub.com

Editor: Leah Huffman
Design and production: Ted Pereda

Printed in China

Preface

In the aviation industry, checklists dramatically reduce the incidence of human error and provide higher safety and success margins. As a licensed pilot, I rely on these checklists for my own safety and that of my passengers, which is why I have introduced similar checklists to use before oral implantology surgical procedures.

Challenges in the cockpit are similar to challenges in the surgical room. Any mistake can lead to drastic consequences. Therefore, just as a safe flight starts with a thorough preflight check (the pilot must check every fastener, inspect every rivet, and evaluate every moving part of the aircraft), implant surgery should start with a thorough presurgery check by the surgeon. Surgeons in the past relied solely on their memory for these checks, but the complexity of the information regarding the procedures today has exceeded our ability as individuals to properly deliver it to our patients in a consistent, correct, and safe manner. Some surgeons hang signs above taps where they wash their hands before surgery reminding them to check that they have the right treatment plan, the correct radiograph, the correct tooth, and even the right patient, but now these signs or post-it notes can be replaced with this very well-organized checklist booklet.

It has short but detailed reminders of all the important steps and their proper sequence that must be followed for the optimal surgical outcome, detailed lists of all instruments needed for most implant-related surgical procedures, postoperative instructions that patients must follow for proper postoperative care that is vital to surgical success, and last but not least, a few lists that provide a clear roadmap to follow in emergency scenarios that might be encountered during or after surgery.

The intent behind this booklet is to provide the implant surgeon (novice and experienced alike) with a tool that provides an extra margin of safety and help in making the surgical procedures (from the instrument setup to the postoperative instructions) run more smoothly and safely by creating a standardized approach and introducing the "culture" of the checklist.

Professionalism and safety come about as a result of an inner drive to do the best job possible, regardless of the circumstances. Competent and superior professionals should perform thorough checks before every procedure—even if no one is watching.

✓	1.1 Diagnostic Data Collection
	Chief complaint of the patient
	Patient's goals and desires
	Health history
	Dental history
	Current and previous medications
	Allergies
	Bisphosphonate treatment (type and amount of time on medication)
	Full-mouth radiographs
	Panoramic radiograph
	Periodontal charting
	Status of existing restorations; etiology of any missing teeth, caries, or fractures
	TMJ evaluation
	Occlusion evaluation
	Soft tissue evaluation (biotype and adequacy of attached keratinized gingiva)
	Oral cancer screening
	Photographs (full face, full face with smile, frontal and lateral views with retractors—with teeth closed and slightly apart, occlusal views)

(cont)

	Impressions and bite registration/facebow, which will be sent to the lab for the fabrication of diagnostic casts, a diagnostic wax-up, and a radiographic template
	Tooth shade
	Shape and size of planned teeth
	Referral to imaging lab for CT scan (radiographic template should be worn during the scan)
	Conversion of the raw CT data to SimPlant (Materialise) or Procera (Nobel Biocare) software protocols if guided surgery is desired

1.2 Risk Factors

Please note that the presence of one risk factor is not necessarily a contraindication to implant treatment. However, the presence of several risk factors represents a high-risk situation or, in some cases, a contraindication to treatment.

✓	General Risk Factors
	Very young or very old age
	Compromised medical condition
	Compromised psychologic condition
	High esthetic demands
	Limited availability for treatment and maintenance appointments
	Smoking habit
	Alcohol abuse
	Temporomandibular disorder
	Periodontal disease
	Etiology of edentulism
	Small jaw opening
	Poor hygiene
	Poor bone density
	Vestibular concavity / Ridge dimensions
	Vertical bone resorption
	Reduced vertical distance between bone crest and opposing tooth
	Mesiodistal dimensions of the edentulous space
	Acute lesions
	Chronic lesions distant from the prospective implant site
	Bony lesions

✓	**Esthetic Risk Factors**
	High maxillary gingival smile line
	Low mandibular gingival smile line
	Scalloped gingiva (high possibility of recession)
	Thin gingiva (high possibility of recession)
	Papillae of adjacent teeth (if thick and short, then "natural regeneration" of the papillae adjacent to the planned implant restoration is facilitated; if long and thin, then complete regeneration is difficult to achieve)
	Form of natural teeth (it is easier to achieve good esthetics with square-shaped teeth than it is with triangular teeth because of the form/architecture of the soft tissue around triangular teeth)
	Shape of interdental contact (the larger the interdental contact surface, the smaller the papillary space and the simpler the papillary regeneration)
	Position of interdental contact (if the contact is less than 5 mm from the bone margin, regeneration of the papilla takes place in practically all cases, but the chances decrease as the distance increases)
	Vestibular concavity
	Existence of adjacent implant (it is difficult to achieve papillary regeneration between two implants because of the absence of a bony papilla [septum] in that situation)
	Vertical bone resorption (this will lead to deep implant placement, unless bone grafting is performed, and to more difficult papillary regeneration)
	Proximal bony peaks (if the proximal bony papillae are absent, soft tissue papillary regeneration will be difficult to achieve)
	High esthetic requirements
	Poor hygiene level
	Unstable provisional restoration

✓	Functional Risk Factors
	Bruxism
	Clenching
	Tongue thrusting
	Large tongue size
	Type of diet
	Posterior position of planned implant (higher stress levels in the posterior region)
	Opposing arch (from more to less favorable, the scenarios are removable implant-supported prosthesis, natural teeth, and fixed implant-supported prosthesis)
	Optimal implant positioning (improper positioning or angulation will lead to bone and soft tissue loss)

✓	Occlusal Risk Factors
	Unbalanced occlusion
	Presence of wear facets
	Posterior bite collapse
	History of cracks and fractures of natural teeth
	Direction of load (if the load on an implant is not directed toward its long axis, a variety of problems will occur, including component failure, prosthetic material failure, and bone loss due to overstress in particular areas, among others)
	Wide occlusal table
	Lateral occlusal contact on the implant-supported prosthesis only

✓	Biomechanical Risk Factors
	Number of implants possible or desired less than the number of roots replaced
	Small implant diameter
	Short implant
	Connection to natural teeth
	Unsplinted implant crowns
	Straight (not tripod) configuration
	Excessive number or size of pontics
	Use of cantilever design
	Implants offset from center of the prosthesis
	Excessively high restoration (unfavorable implant length-to-crown height ratio)
	Unsatisfactory primary implant stability
	Lack of passive prosthetic fit
	Pier abutment
	Mandibular flexion
	Immediate loading

1.3 CT Scan Evaluation

✓	Mandibular CT Scan
	Evaluate the position of the inferior alveolar nerve (distance from the alveolar crest, path, and diameter).
	Assess the position of the mental foramen/nerve.
	Check for the existence and the extensiveness of the mental nerve loop.
	Watch for the incisive mandibular canal (length and distance from the crestal ridge).
	Take account of any possible undercuts (sublabial, subbuccal, submandibular fossa, and subdigastric fossa).
	Evaluate the topography of the alveolar ridge/bone (look for crestal ridge irregularities).
	Locate the accessory lingual foramina and determine their distance from the crestal ridge.
	Appraise the curvature of the teeth adjacent to the planned osteotomy site(s).
	Evaluate the bone density (in general and at the planned implant site[s] in particular).
	Check for any possible pathologies in the bone or in the nerve canals.
	Watch for possible root remnants at the intended implant site(s).
	Evaluate for adequate alveolar dimensions (in height and width) for single or multiple implant placement.

✓	Maxillary CT Scan
	Evaluate the position of the incisive foramen/canal relative to the anterior alveolar crest.
	Appraise the vault shape of the palate to estimate the location of the greater palatine artery and nerve.
	Check for undercuts (sublabial and subbuccal).
	Assess the topography of the alveolar ridge/bone.
	Gauge the curvature of the teeth adjacent to the planned osteotomy site(s).
	Watch for possible root remnants at the intended implant site(s).
	Evaluate the bone density (in general and at the planned implant site[s] in particular).
	Check for any pathologies in the bone or in the nerve canals.
	Verify adequate alveolar dimensions (in height and width) for single or multiple implant placement.
	Assess the distance available for implant placement under the sinus floor.
	Gauge the distance available for implant placement under the nasal floor.
	Check the sinus for existence of septa.
	Evaluate the sinus for existence of soft tissue pathologies.

Please note that soft tissue anatomical structures (eg, gingival thickness and quality and the lingual nerve) cannot be evaluated on the CT scan; however, they are important to the overall success of the surgical phase of the implant treatment.

1.4 Immediate Loading Guidelines

✓	Single Implant Cases
	Rule out the existence of any parafunctions (see the Functional Risk Factors Checklist, page 11).
	Confirm initial stability ≥ 40 Ncm of torque.
	Determine that bone has greater than D3 density (immediate loading should not be performed in soft bone even in the presence of high initial stability).
	Place the provisional crown out of the occlusion.
	Do not perform immediate loading distal to the first molar (in second molar area).
	Do not use short implants for single immediate loading cases. Check implant-crown ratio (minimum implant length of 9 mm when performing immediate loading).
	Instruct the patient to follow a soft diet for a minimum of 8 weeks.
	Perform immediate loading only in cooperative patients.

✓	Multiple Implant Cases
The rules below are to be followed in addition to the rules for single implant immediate loading.	
	Splint the provisional crowns.
	Keep the pontic as short as possible.
	Do not use a cantilever design.
	Ensure balanced occlusion of natural teeth (ie, no contact on the partial immediate-load prosthesis).
	Confirm that an adequate number of implants are being placed.
	Use a screw-retained provisional prosthesis (if possible).
	Ensure maintenance of good oral hygiene.

✓	Full-Arch Implant Cases
The rules below are to be followed in addition to the rules for single and multiple implant immediate loading.	
	Place a minimum of 5 implants in the mandible and 7 in the maxilla.
	Implants should be evenly spaced.
	Confirm a passive fit of the implant prosthesis.
	Ensure balanced occlusion.
	Establish optimal implant positioning (angular and axial inclination).

Things to consider in all three scenarios: opposing dentition and the patient's size, age, sex, and diet.

✓	1.5 Treatment Plan Development
	Review the patient's health history for any possible limitations (eg, diabetes or recent radiotherapy).
	Analyze all radiographs (periapical and panoramic).
	Examine photographs to determine soft tissue quality and quantity, arch relationship, and bite.
	Study the diagnostic wax-up to evaluate occlusion, arch relationship, soft tissue characteristics, and the available vertical and horizontal spaces of occlusion.
	On the CT scan, evaluate the volume of the available alveolar bone for implant placement, anatomical landmarks, bone density, any bone defects that may require bone augmentation, and any possible pathologies (see CT Scan Evaluation Checklist, page 13).
	Evaluate any possible risk factors (see Risk Factors Checklist, page 9).
	Consider special factors such as template use; immediate or sequenced treatment protocol; prosthesis type; implant type, number, length, diameter, position, and angulation; provisional prosthesis; and prognosis.
	Consult with the laboratory regarding the prosthetic design and cost.
	Develop goal-oriented treatment plans. A minimum of 2 treatment plans should be presented.
	Schedule a case presentation visit with the patient.

✓	1.6 Case Presentation Visit
	Present the treatment plan options using patient education models, patient education software, treatment planning software (eg, SimPlant), and a diagnostic wax-up.
	Review the limitations and risk factors.
	Estimate the treatment length (both surgical and prosthetic phases).
	Describe the provisional prosthesis.
	Describe the definitive prosthesis.
	Explain the required medications.
	Discuss the possible complications.
	Review the maintenance requirements (professional and home care protocol).
	Explain the breakdown of fees.
	Present the financial options.
	Acquire informed consent (if the patient approves one of the treatment plans).
	After the visit, distribute a treatment plan confirmation letter to the patient, emphasizing the treatment plans discussed as well as all of the above points.

✓	2.1 Basic Implant Placement
	Acquire consent. Give the patient enough time to go over consent forms and the opportunity to express any questions or concerns, and then obtain a signature. More than one consent form may be needed (eg, one consent form for the extraction procedures and one for the oral sedation, if utilized).
	Prescribe medication. Antibiotics, an anti-inflammatory drug, an analgesic, and an antibacterial mouthrinse are recommended.
	Administer anesthesia. Local anesthesia is usually adequate; however, intravenous or oral sedation may be used in addition.
	Elevate a full-thickness flap (two-wall, three-wall, or envelope flap as needed) or use a tissue punch if placement with a flapless technique is selected.
	Make final measurements of available bone to select the optimal implant size (diameter and length) and implant positioning according to the dimensions of the actual alveolar bone. If no CT scan was obtained, actual bone dimensions may be different from those measured on radiographs.
	Evaluate the thickness of the tissue in the crestal area. (This will affect the depth of implant placement as well as the length of the healing abutment in case of a one-stage placement protocol.)
	Place the surgical template (if one was prepared before the surgery).
	Perform the initial osteotomy. Start with a small round drill to create an entry point in a narrow crest or start immediately with the initial pilot drill (2.0 mm). Always use copious irrigation with refrigerated sterile water or sterile saline.

(cont)

	Take a radiograph with a parallel pin in place. The radiograph will reveal the osteotomy direction and position in relation to certain anatomical landmarks. At this stage, it is usually not too late to change the direction and the position of the osteotomy. Remember to tie a length of floss around the parallel pin to simplify its retrieval if necessary (Fig 1).

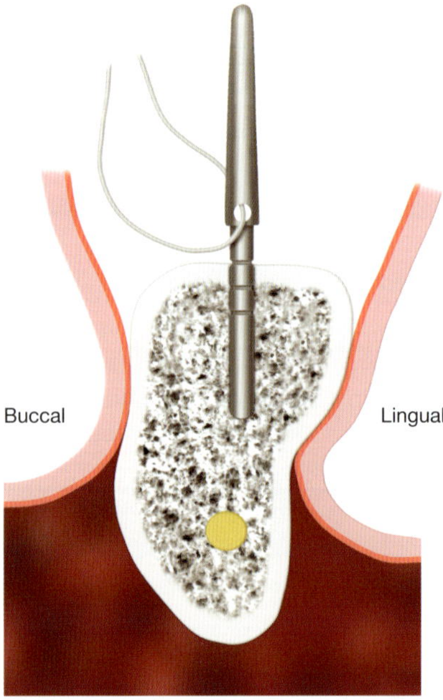

Fig 1

	Continue the osteotomy (once satisfied with its direction and position on the radiograph) per the implant's size and diameter and the bone type.
	Perform thread forming (tapping). This is indicated in dense bone only. Use a high-torque handpiece or hand ratchet. The thread former/tapping drill should feed without pressure (use slow speed with irrigation). When done, set the motor in the reverse mode and back the thread former out; do not pull on the thread former.

(cont)

	Irrigate the osteotomy site and use suction to remove any debris (but do not blow air into the osteotomy site).
	Place the implant to the desired level with the ratchet or handpiece. Do not overtighten the implant, and do not touch the implant with gloves. Initial stability should be obtained. The implant can be placed with or without irrigation.
	Take a final radiograph for the patient's records.
	Place a healing abutment for a single-stage protocol, a cover screw for a two-stage protocol, or a definitive prosthetic abutment for an immediate loading protocol.
	Place the sutures. Gore-Tex (W. L. Gore) or Vicryl (Ethicon) suture materials are recommended.
	Provide postoperative instructions. The patient should be given instructions regarding hygiene, diet, and medications (see Postoperative Instructions for Implant Placement/GBR Checklist, page 59).
	If a provisional prosthesis is to be used, it should not exert any pressure on the implant site during the healing phase.
	Schedule a 2-week follow-up appointment for a postoperative checkup and suture removal.

✓	2.2 Socket Grafting and Ridge Preservation
	Acquire consent. Give the patient enough time to go over consent forms and the opportunity to express any questions or concerns, and then obtain a signature. More than one consent form may be needed (eg, one consent form for the extraction procedures and one for the oral sedation, if utilized).
	Prescribe medication. Antibiotics, an anti-inflammatory drug, an analgesic, and an antibacterial mouthrinse are recommended.
	Administer anesthesia. Local anesthesia is usually adequate; however, intravenous or oral sedation may be used in addition.
	Make a sulcular incision around the tooth to be extracted using a 15C blade. If the root to be extracted is below the crestal bone level, reflection of a small envelope flap is recommended.
	Perform atraumatic extraction (using periotomes, luxators, and, if necessary, root tip forceps). The periotomes should be used mainly on the mesial and distal of the tooth to be extracted. When using forceps, limit the buccolingual movement to minimize the possibility of fracturing the buccal plate. A piezotome machine can also be used for atraumatic extraction, if available.
	Perform thorough debridement or degranulation of the socket, especially if chronic infection exists, using small Lucas curettes. The socket grafting procedure should not be performed if an acute infection is present.
	Use a periodontal probe to identify any natural dehiscence or fenestrations on the buccal wall. If detected, these openings or defects must be covered with a membrane following flap reflection.
	Prepare the graft material by hydrating it with sterile saline or the patient's blood to achieve a workable consistency, and then transfer the graft to the socket using a periosteal elevator or bone grafting syringe.
	Pack the socket with bone graft material up to the crestal bone level. Allograft of a small particle size is preferred because it usually takes a long time for xenograft or alloplast materials to resorb.

(cont)

	Do not condense the bone graft material too firmly because it is necessary for the osseous blood in the socket to flow freely between the particulates of the graft material. The bone graft material prevents the collapse of the buccal socket wall and acts only as a matrix or scaffold for bone growth in the extraction area; therefore, the blood in the socket must moisten the graft material.
	Place a piece of collagen resorbable membrane or plug on the top of the graft material, which should have been cut to an appropriate size.
	Place a criss-cross suture over the collagen dressing. Primary closure is not possible after extraction and is not necessary with the use of a membrane and an adequate number of sutures. The goal is not to close the socket but to keep the membrane in place. Gore-Tex (W. L. Gore) or Vicryl (Ethicon) suture materials are recommended.
	Provide postoperative instructions. The patient should be given instructions regarding hygiene, diet, and medications (see Post-operative Instructions for Socket Grafting Checklist, page 60).
	If a provisional prosthesis is to be used, an ovate pontic design is preferred, but it should not exert excessive pressure on the grafted area during the healing phase.
	Schedule a 2-week follow-up appointment for a postoperative checkup and suture removal.

2.3 Second-Stage Surgery

After an appropriate healing period (usually 2 to 9 months depending on the initial stability and bone density type), the implant is exposed and a healing abutment (permucosal extension) placed in order to create a permucosal seal around the implant and achieve optimal soft tissue architecture and emergence profile around the future implant prosthesis. Three techniques are available for this exposure: the soft tissue punch, an incision with a scalpel, and the Palacci techniques.

A soft tissue punch or a combination of an incision followed by a tissue punch can be used when the planned prosthesis is a removable (ie, bar-overdenture and locator-overdenture prostheses) or a fixed-detachable prosthesis (ie, high-water and spark-erosion prostheses). However, when the planned prosthesis is an implant-supported fixed prosthesis (ie, crown and partial denture type) in the esthetic zone, then the author recommends the Palacci techniques of soft tissue manipulation for achieving better soft tissue architecture and fuller papillae around the implant crown.

✓	Tissue Punch and Incision Techniques
	Use a scalpel to make an incision, incorporating a flap if you cannot see exactly where the implant is. If you are sure where the cover screw is or can at least locate the center of it with a scalpel (this is possible when the soft tissue is thin), you can use a soft tissue punch (either disposable or on a handpiece).
	Remove the cover screw.
	Flush the inside of the implant with Peridex (3M ESPE), using a 3-mL syringe, and then blow dry.
	Place the appropriate healing abutment. (Healing abutments come in a variety of heights. You should use the one that extends 1 to 2 mm above the soft tissue level. They also have varying widths, with some as wide as the implant [cylindric] and some wider than the implant's platform. Unless the implant is in the esthetic zone and the biotype is thin, you should use the wider one because it provides a better tissue environment for the placement of the impression post or the definitive prosthetic abutment.)

(cont)

	Place two or more sutures if a flap was necessary; no sutures are needed if you used a tissue punch directly.
	Remove the sutures 2 weeks postoperative.
	Take the impression 2 to 3 weeks after suture removal; if no sutures were needed, take the impression 1 to 2 weeks after exposure of the implant.
	Perform immediate loading only in cooperative patients.

Figures 1 and 2 illustrate both techniques described above.

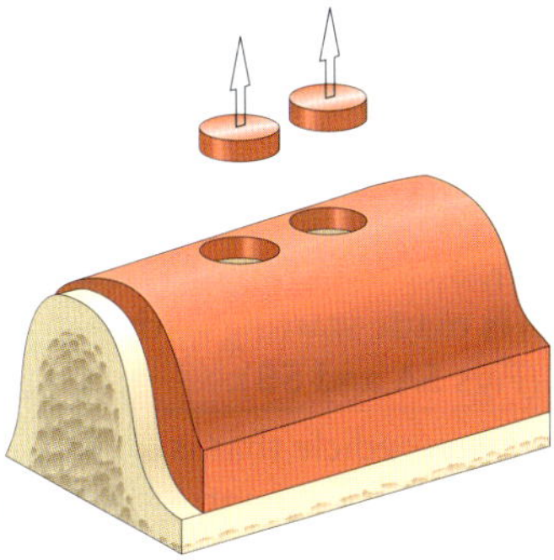

Fig 1

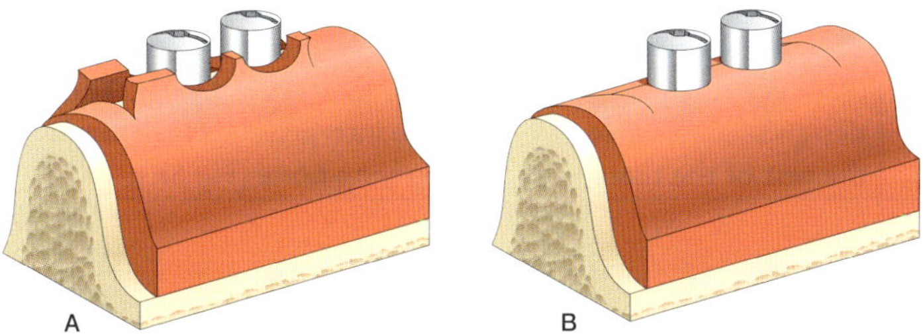

Fig 2 A B

✓	Palacci Techniques
Creating papillae around an implant	
	Elevate a full-thickness flap in the buccal direction, then make a T-shaped incision and slide both sides of the flap laterally to fill the space between the abutment and the adjacent teeth (Fig 3).
Creating a papilla between two implants	
	Elevate a full-thickness flap in the buccal direction, then make semilunar bevel incisions (distal to mesial) to allow two pedicles to rotate with a 90-degree angulation (Fig 4A), creating a central papilla (Fig 4B).
Creating papillae between implants or between an implant and a natural tooth	
	Elevate a full-thickness flap in the buccal direction, then make a semilunar bevel incision in the flap in relation to each implant. The first incision is made starting at the distal aspect of the most mesial implant (Figs 5A and 5B).
	The incision creates a pedicle that is rotated 90 degrees toward the mesial aspect of the abutment. The semilunar bevel incision must be extended far enough to allow the pedicle to be rotated and placed in the interproximal area without tension. Figures 5C and 5D illustrate the occlusal view of pedicle rotation.
	Place the first single suture at the mesial aspect at the releasing incision, followed by three horizontal mattress sutures starting buccally and running to the palatal aspect and back. This suture design stabilizes the pedicle in the interproximal area and adapts the rest of the tissue to the underlying bone (Fig 5E).

(cont)

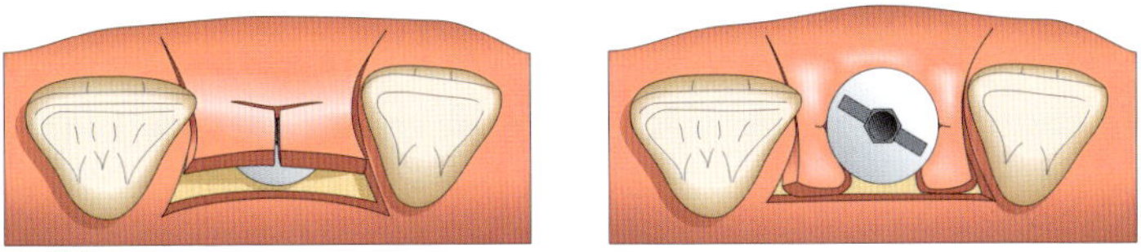

A B

Fig 3

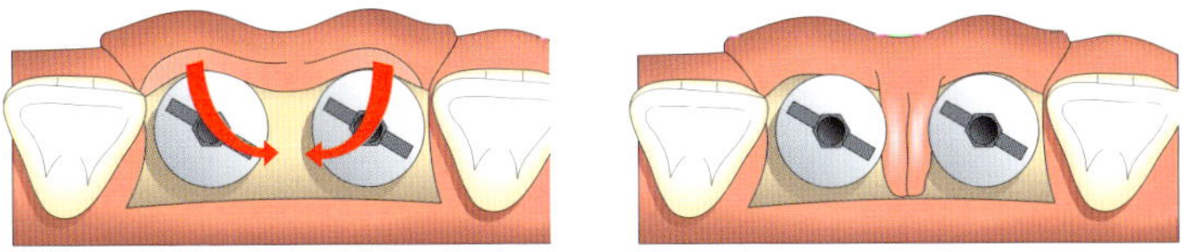

A B

Fig 4

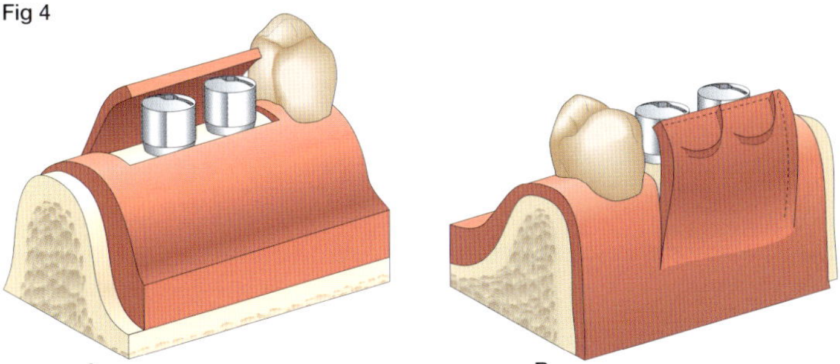

A B

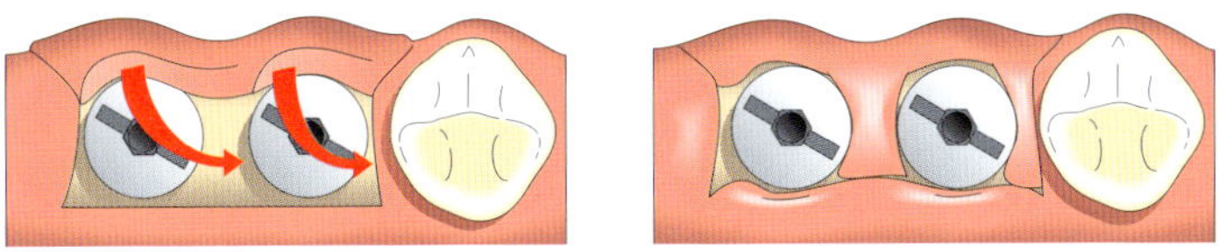

C D

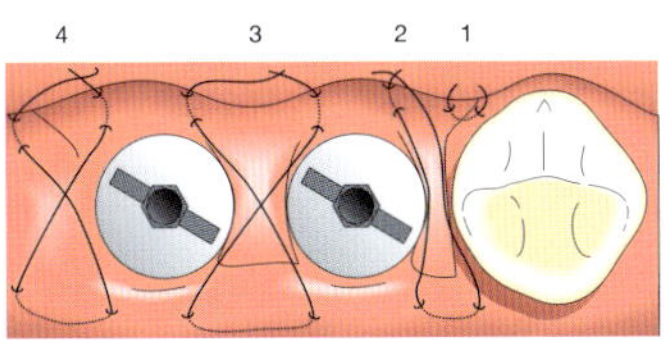

Fig 5 E

2.4 Crestal Sinus Elevation

This procedure is indicated when there is no less than 5 mm of available bone under the sinus floor and yet a deficiency of up to 4 mm for implant placement (Fig 1A). In order to raise the sinus floor more than 4 mm using this procedure, the author highly recommends incorporating a sinuscope to monitor the progress of the procedure.

The technique described below is the Al-Faraje technique for sinus elevation using a crestal approach.

✓	Crestal Sinus Elevation
	Develop a treatment plan after a thorough clinical examination and review of the patient's CT scan. (See the Treatment Plan Development Checklist, page 17.)
	Acquire consent. Give the patient enough time to go over consent forms and the opportunity to express any questions or concerns, and then obtain a signature. More than one consent form may be needed (eg, one consent form for the implant placement procedures, one for the crestal sinus elevation, and one for the oral sedation, if utilized).
	Prescribe medication. Antibiotics, an anti-inflammatory drug, an analgesic, and an antibacterial mouthrinse are recommended.
	Administer anesthesia. Local anesthesia is usually adequate; however, intravenous or oral sedation may be used in addition.
	Gain access to the crestal bone via a soft tissue punch or a full-thickness flap.
	Use the pilot drill all the way to the sinus floor (but be careful not to perforate it) (Fig 1B).
	Take a radiograph to check the positioning and angulation of the pilot osteotomy and to verify close proximity to but not penetration of the sinus floor.
	Use all drills (or implant osteotomes) necessary to enlarge the osteotomy sufficiently for the intended implant diameter (Fig 1C). (Note that all drills or implant osteotomes must stop slightly short of the sinus floor at this stage.)

(cont)

	Select the sinus osteotome (with a concave tip and stoppers [Salvin]) that matches the apical diameter of the osteotomy created and place its stopper at a distance from its tip that matches the intended implant's length (ie, it will be up to 4 mm longer than the osteotomy) (Fig 1D).
	Gently tap the floor of the sinus with a mallet to cause a green-stick fracture, then slowly introduce the sinus osteotome until the stopper reaches the crestal bone (Fig 1E).
	Remove the sinus osteotome and introduce a 10 × 10-mm collagen wound dressing (eg, Oratape or OraPlug [Salvin]) into the osteotomy. Then introduce a small amount of bone graft material (0.25 mL is usually adequate; the author prefers allograft) into the osteotomy (Fig 1F).
	Place the implant (Fig 1G).
	Place the cover screw or healing abutment. (The healing abutment should be chosen for good initial stability and bone density.)
	Provide postoperative instructions. The patient should be given instructions regarding hygiene, diet, and medications (see Postoperative Instructions for Sinus Elevation Procedure Checklist, page 63).
	If a provisional prosthesis is to be used, it should not exert any pressure on the implant site during the healing phase.
	Schedule a 2-week follow-up appointment for a postoperative checkup and suture removal.

(cont)

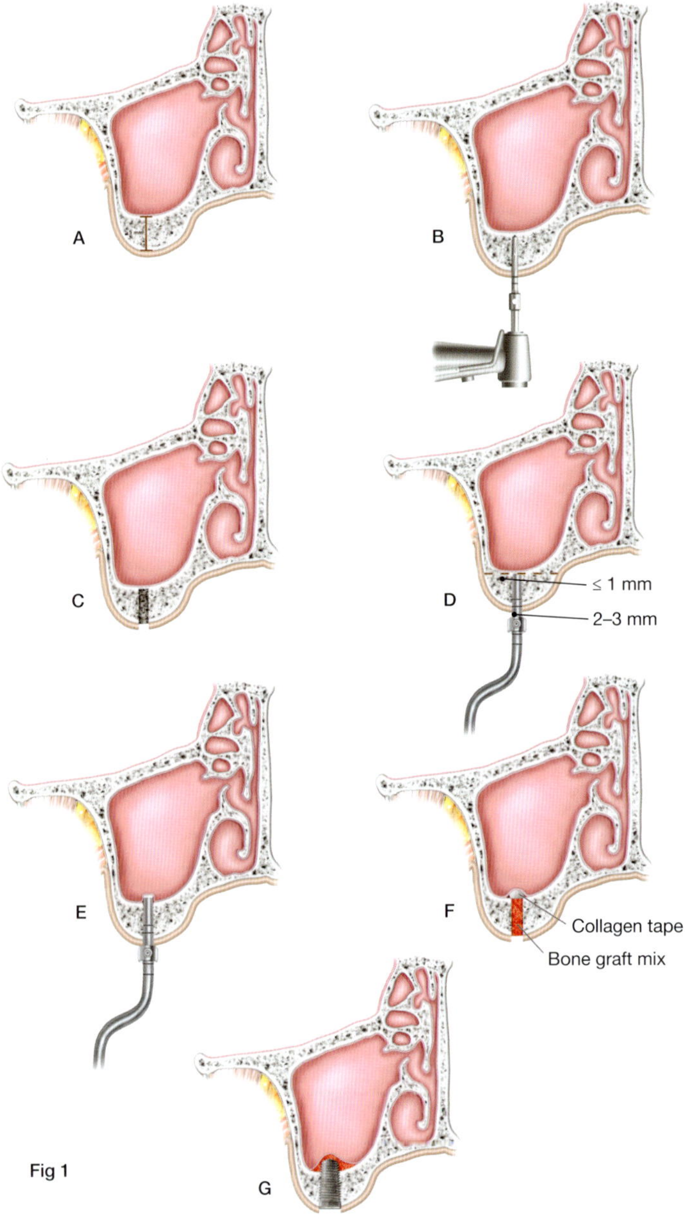

Fig 1

2.5 GBR Protocol Using Particulate Bone Graft Materials and Either a Resorbable or Nonresorbable Membrane

☐	Acquire consent. Give the patient enough time to go over consent forms and the opportunity to express any questions or concerns, and then obtain a signature. More than one consent form may be needed (eg, one consent form for extraction procedures and one for the oral sedation, if utilized).
☐	Prescribe medication. Antibiotics, an anti-inflammatory drug, an analgesic, and an antibacterial mouthrinse are recommended.
☐	Prescribe anesthesia. Local anesthesia is usually adequate; however, intravenous or oral sedation may be used in addition.
☐	Make a midcrestal and two releasing incisions approximately 1 to 2 teeth away from the planned graft site on each side.

Notes:
- Blade no. 12C is the blade of choice for most cases.
- In the maxilla, the midcrestal incision can be placed slightly more palatally because the palatal flap cannot be stretched.

☐	Clean the bone of any periosteum or muscle attachments using a back-action chisel (ie, Rhodes Chisel, Salvin).
☐	If GBR is being performed with simultaneous implant placement, place the implant(s).

Notes:
- Place the implant in the optimal position buccolingually and apicocoronally despite the deficient bone volume (because the deficient areas will be augmented with bone graft material around the exposed areas of the implant).
- The apical portion of the implant should be completely embedded in bone.
- The implant should have good initial stability.

(cont)

<table>
<tr><td></td><td>Perforate (ie, decorticate) for bleeding points. This is a very important step. Create approximately 10 holes with a small round diamond bur. If an implant has been placed, the bleeding points are created around and apical to the implant.</td></tr>
<tr><td></td><td>Place tenting screws on the buccal plate and on the crest if needed.</td></tr>
<tr><td colspan="2">Notes:
· Tenting screws are to be used when more than a 2-mm gain in width is required.
· Usually 2 to 3 tenting screws are adequate.</td></tr>
<tr><td></td><td>Harvest autogenous bone (eg, from the tuberosity). There are a variety of instruments available to harvest bone intraorally such as rongeurs and trephine drills.</td></tr>
<tr><td></td><td>If a nonresorbable membrane is being used, fix the membrane buccally with screws or tacks before adding the graft material.</td></tr>
<tr><td></td><td>Add the autogenous bone layer.</td></tr>
<tr><td></td><td>Add the xenograft material. If no autogenous bone is to be used, then use an allograft and xenograft (50/50) mix.</td></tr>
<tr><td></td><td>Affix the membrane on the crest or the lingual/palatal side if a nonresorbable membrane is being used.</td></tr>
<tr><td colspan="2">Notes:
· If a resorbable membrane is being used, place two layers. There is usually no need to affix the membrane with tacks or screws because these membranes usually are adhesive enough to stay exactly where intended.
· When a nonresorbable membrane is used, the border of the membrane should be well under the flap away from the incision line.
· When a nonresorbable membrane is used, it should be 1 mm away from adjacent teeth on the crest.</td></tr>
</table>

(cont)

	Release the flap for tension-free closure using a scalpel to score the periosteum and then Metzenbaum scissors if needed to release the muscle layer. If the amount of ridge augmentation is substantial, muscle layer release is highly recommended for tension-free incision line closure.
	Suture the flap under no tension.
Notes: · Gore-Tex (W. L. Gore) is the suture material of choice. Use 4-0 or 5-0 depending on the thickness of the soft tissue. · Sutures must remain in place for 2 weeks. · The waiting period for bone maturation is 9 to 12 months. · The patient should not wear an interim prosthesis in the GBR area for 2 weeks.	
	Take a radiograph for the patient's records.
	Provide postoperative instructions. The patient should be given instructions regarding hygiene, diet, and medications (see Postoperative Instructions for Implant Placement/GBR Checklist, page 59).
	Schedule a 2-week follow-up appointment for a postoperative checkup and suture removal.

✓	2.6 GBR Protocol Using rhBMP-2/ACS and Titanium Mesh
	Acquire consent. Give the patient enough time to go over consent forms and the opportunity to express any questions or concerns, and then obtain a signature. More than one consent form may be needed (eg, one consent form for extraction procedures and one for the oral sedation, if utilized).
	Prescribe medication. Antibiotics, an anti-inflammatory drug, an analgesic, and an antibacterial mouthrinse are recommended.
	Administer anesthesia. Local anesthesia is usually adequate; however, intravenous or oral sedation may be used in addition.
	Make a midcrestal and two releasing incisions approximately 1 to 2 teeth away from the planned graft site on each side.
Notes: · Blade no. 12C is the blade of choice for most cases. · In the maxilla, the midcrestal incision can be placed slightly more palatally because the palatal flap cannot be stretched.	
	Clean the bone of any periosteum or muscle attachments using a back-action chisel (ie, Rhodes Chisel, Salvin).
	If GBR is being performed with simultaneous implant placement, place the implant(s).
Notes: · Place the implant in the optimal position buccolingually and apicocoronally despite the deficient bone volume (because the deficient areas will be augmented with bone graft material around the exposed areas of the implant). · The apical portion of the implant should be completely embedded in bone. · The implant should have good initial stability.	

(cont)

<table>
<tr><td></td><td>Perforate (ie, decorticate) for bleeding points. This is a very important step. Create approximately 10 holes with a small round diamond bur. If an implant has been placed, the bleeding points are created around and apical to the implant.</td></tr>
<tr><td></td><td>Apply the rhBMP-2/ACS material per the manufacturer guidelines (xenograft material can be added to the BMP collagen sponge).</td></tr>
<tr><td></td><td>Affix the titanium mesh using fixation screws.</td></tr>
<tr><td colspan="2">Notes:
· The border of the titanium mesh should be well under the flap (there should be no mesh directly under the incision lines).
· On the crest, there should be a distance of 2 mm between the titanium mesh and adjacent teeth.</td></tr>
<tr><td></td><td>Release the flap for tension-free closure using a scalpel to score the periosteum and then Metzenbaum scissors to release the muscle layer.</td></tr>
<tr><td></td><td>Suture the flap under no tension.</td></tr>
<tr><td colspan="2">Notes:
· Gore-Tex (W. L. Gore) is the suture material of choice. Use 4-0 or 5-0 depending on the thickness of the soft tissue.
· Sutures must remain in place for 2 weeks.
· The waiting period for bone maturation is 9 months.
· The patient should not wear an interim prosthesis in the GBR area for 2 weeks.</td></tr>
<tr><td></td><td>Take a radiograph for the patient's records.</td></tr>
<tr><td></td><td>Provide postoperative instructions. The patient should be given instructions regarding hygiene, diet, and medications (see Post-operative Instructions for Implant Placement/GBR Checklist, page 59).</td></tr>
<tr><td></td><td>Schedule a 2-week follow-up appointment for a postoperative checkup and suture removal.</td></tr>
</table>

2.7 Alveolar Ridge Expansion Using the Split-Ridge Technique

Develop a treatment plan after a thorough clinical exam and review of the patient's CT scan to determine whether the split-ridge technique may be used. (See the Treatment Plan Development Checklist, page 17.) This procedure is indicated in the anterior maxilla with certain types of ridge resorption and only between the maxillary sinuses. Ridge splitting directly below the sinuses is not recommended. (Figures 1 and 5A show a ridge resorption pattern that is a candidate for the ridge splitting technique, while Fig 2 shows a pattern that may not be treated using this technique.)

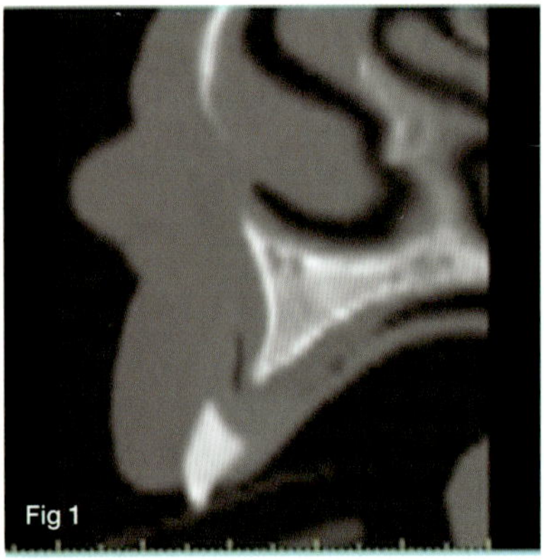
Fig 1

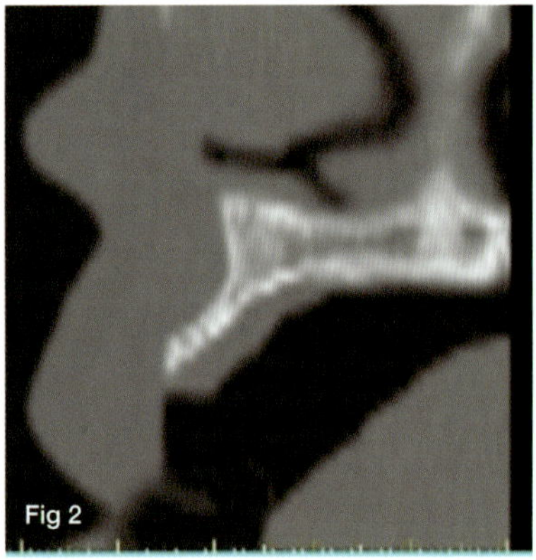
Fig 2

Note:
The author is introducing a new classification for natural resorption patterns of the alveolar bone in which resorption pattern is divided into 2 forms (Fig 3). Current classifications state that after tooth loss the alveolar bone gradually loses width until it is severe and then height loss begins, but the author rather argues that after the initial width loss, the resorption pattern takes on 2 different formats: severe width loss along the entire alveolar bone (see Figs 2, 3D, and 3I) or severe width loss only in the crestal half of the alveolar bone with a good amount of alveolar bone width remaining in the apical half (see Figs 1, 3C, and 3H). It is important to be aware of these 2 different patterns and be able to distinguish between them on the CT scan during the CT evaluation and treatment planning stage because the resorption pattern will dictate the bone grafting procedures required to augment the ridge.

(cont)

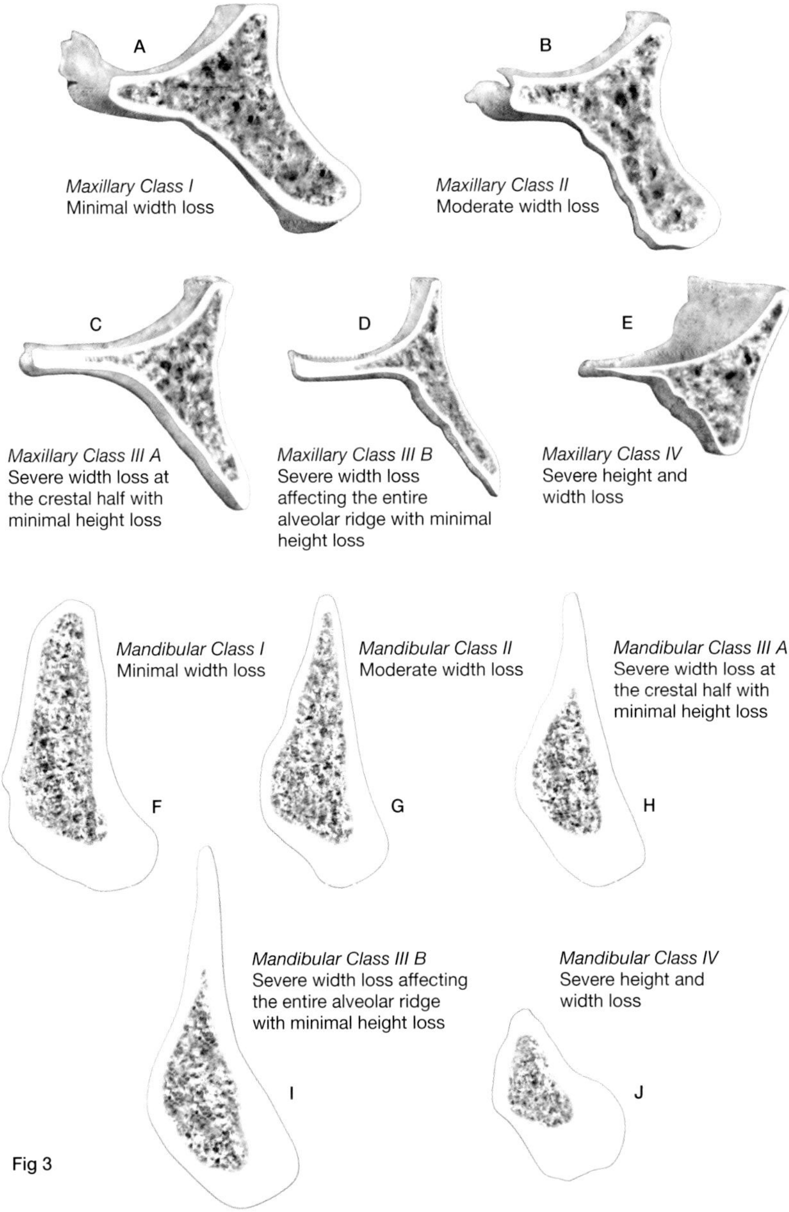
A
Maxillary Class I
Minimal width loss
B
Maxillary Class II
Moderate width loss
C
Maxillary Class III A
Severe width loss at the crestal half with minimal height loss
D
Maxillary Class III B
Severe width loss affecting the entire alveolar ridge with minimal height loss
E
Maxillary Class IV
Severe height and width loss
Mandibular Class I
Minimal width loss
F
Mandibular Class II
Moderate width loss
G
Mandibular Class III A
Severe width loss at the crestal half with minimal height loss
H
Mandibular Class III B
Severe width loss affecting the entire alveolar ridge with minimal height loss
I
Mandibular Class IV
Severe height and width loss
J

Fig 3

	Acquire consent. Give the patient enough time to go over consent forms and the opportunity to express any questions or concerns, and then obtain a signature. More than one consent form may be needed (eg, implant placement, sandwich bone grafting, and oral sedation, if used).
	Prescribe medication. Antibiotics, an anti-inflammatory drug, an analgesic, and an antibacterial mouthrinse are recommended.
	Administer anesthesia. Local anesthesia is usually adequate; however, intravenous or oral sedation may be used in addition.
	Reflect a full-thickness flap. The flap should be large enough to allow visualization of the alveolar bone's width, shape, and trajectory. On each side, the flap should extend approximately 10 mm distal to the area to be split (Fig 5B).
	Perform an alveoloplasty to flatten the crestal ridge. A minimum amount of bony ridge should be removed to achieve the goal of the alveoloplasty while avoiding the placement of short implants and maintaining a safe distance from the nasal floor.
	Perform the initial osteotomy. A no. 699 XXL bur is used to the full depth of its cutting part to create a longitudinal cut in the middle of the alveolar crest. This step should be done with great care to prevent perforations of the labial or palatal plates. (Alternatively, a Piezotome can be used to perform this part of the procedure.) Always use copious irrigation with refrigerated sterile water or sterile saline. The bur should not be inserted deeper than 10 mm.
	Make osseous releasing incisions (optional). If the cortex is thick, a round diamond bur is used to make osseous releasing incisions (one horizontal and two vertical). The cuts should be in the cortex layer only and should not extend to the cancellous bone.
	Continue expansion. The expanding chisel is introduced into the osteotomy. The expansion chisels can be purchased from a variety of sources and usually come in 3-, 4-, 5-, and 6-mm diameters (Figs 4 and 5C). It is important to note that if more than two chisels are used, the maxillary bone will lose its elasticity, in which case

(cont)

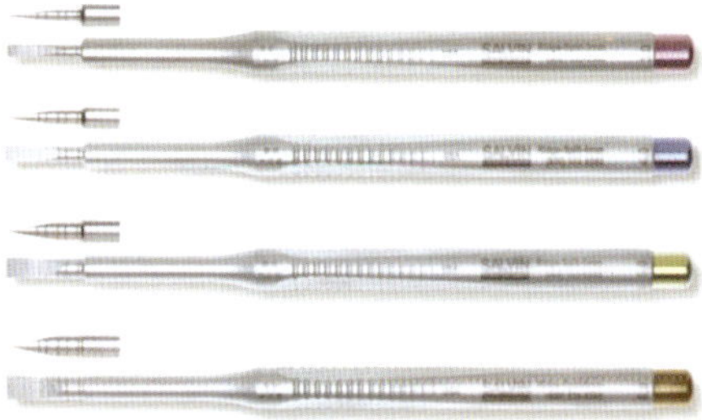

Fig 4

	simultaneous implant placement is not possible and rather a two-step protocol with delayed implant placement (in 4 to 5 months) must be followed. However, if only the first 1 or 2 chisels are used, then the next step is implant placement. Placement of the implants immediately after the ridge-splitting procedure is preferable to prevent any collapse that might occur in the two-stage protocol. Chisels must be used to the entire length of the planned implants.
	Place the implant. The osteotomies must be under-prepped (stop short of the implants' diameter), then the implants are placed (Figs 5D and 5E).
	Place bone graft material between the implants, and then cover the entire expansion area with a collagen membrane (eg, Oratape, Salvin).
	Suture the flap after release of the periosteal layer for tension-free primary closure (Fig 5F).
	Take a final radiograph for the patient's records.
	Deliver the provisional restoration. After the ridge augmentation procedure, the old removable prosthesis cannot be used because of the change in the alveolar ridge dimensions, so fabrication of a new removable provisional restoration is indicated.
	Provide postoperative instructions. The patient should be given instructions regarding hygiene, diet, and medications (see Postoperative Instructions for Implant Placement/GBR Checklist, page 59).

(cont)

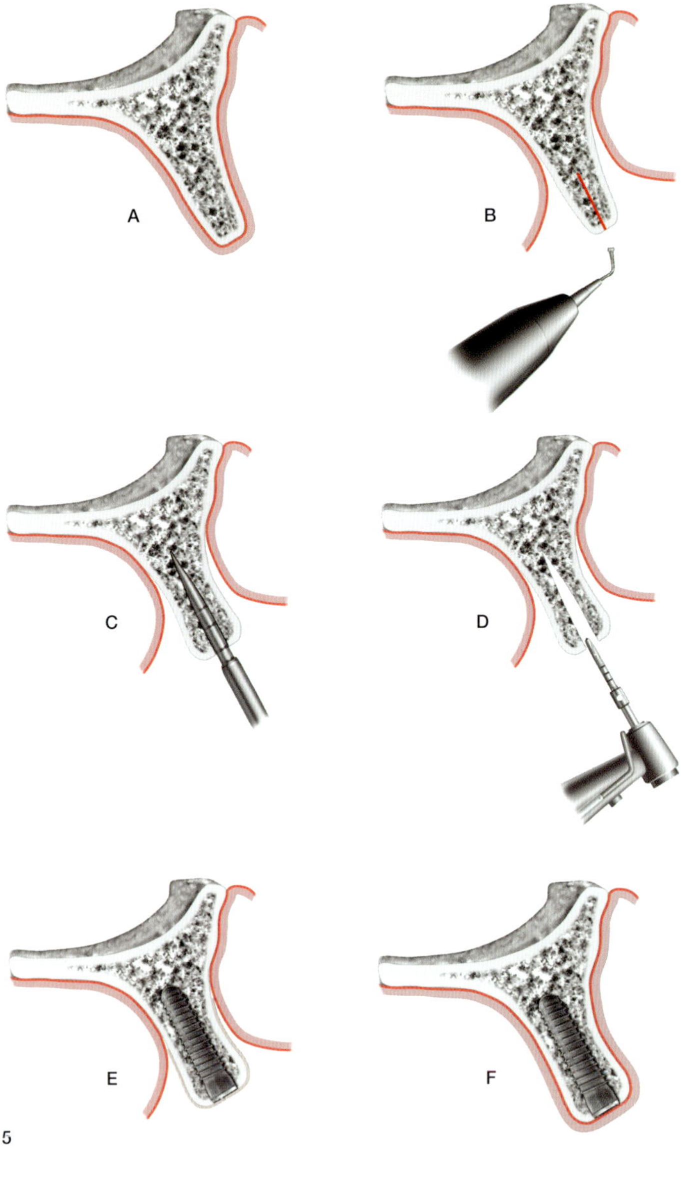

Fig 5

✓	2.8 Grafting Using Allograft Block
	Develop a treatment plan after a thorough clinical exam and review of the patient's CT scan. (See the Treatment Plan Development Checklist, page 17.) The shape of the bone loss pattern and the architecture of the soft tissue must be evaluated to verify that the edentulous area is a candidate for block grafting.
	Acquire consent. Give the patient enough time to go over consent forms and the opportunity to express any questions or concerns, and then obtain a signature. More than one consent form may be needed (eg, one consent form for the oral sedation and one for simultaneous soft tissue grafting).
	Prescribe medication. Antibiotics, an anti-inflammatory drug, an analgesic, and an antibacterial mouthrinse are recommended.
	Administer anesthesia. Infiltration and/or block anesthesia in addition to oral sedation are recommended; however, the clinician might elect to use intravenous sedation instead of oral.

(cont)

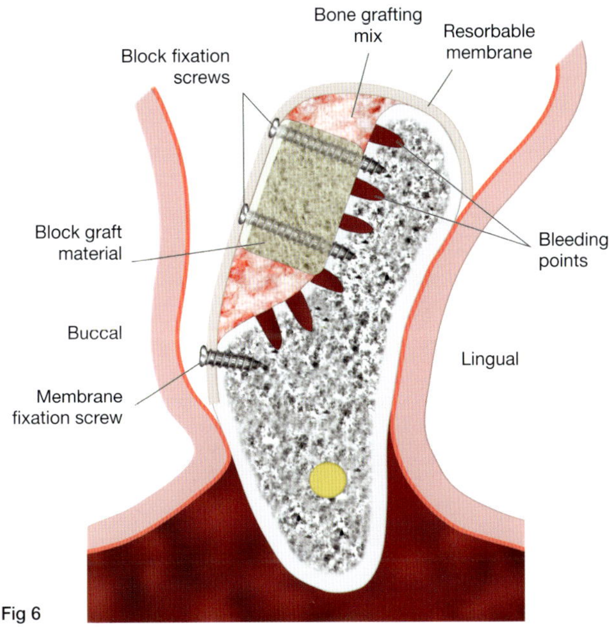

Fig 6

	Make the incisions and reflect a full-thickness flap. The mid-crestal and releasing oblique incisions should be large enough and approximately 15 mm mesial and distal to the planned block borders to allow for tension-free closure at the conclusion of the block grafting procedure.
	Prepare the receptor site. Using a large alveoloplasty bur, prepare an inlay site, and then create perforations using a small round or 1.1-mm straight bur to ensure bleeding from the cancellous bone layer (ie, the buccal wall is decorticated).
	Hydrate the block graft. The block graft should be submerged in sterile saline for approximately 5 minutes.

✓	**Tips for Block Fixation**
	The lag screw technique should be followed.
	A minimum of 2 screws is required to prevent any block movement or rotation.
	A small round bur is used to countersink the cortical layer so the heads of the fixation screws will be flush with the cortical bone surface. This will minimize the chances for soft tissue perforation or dehiscence during the healing period from the otherwise extruding screw heads.
	Overtightening of the screws should be avoided.
	The 2 screws should not be too close to each other to avoid fracture in that region of the block.
	It is important to engage the cortical plate of the opposing side of the recipient site; therefore, short fixation screws should not be used.
	Exposed screw tips on the lingual or palatal side can be cut with a fissure bur.
	After fixation of the block graft, the block edges and corners should be checked for any sharp areas, and if any are encountered, they should be smoothed with a large round diamond bur.

✓	2.9 Sinus Augmentation Using the Lateral Window Technique
	Develop a treatment plan after a thorough clinical exam and review of the patient's CT scan. (See the Treatment Plan Development Checklist, page 17.) The sinus must be evaluated for any possible soft tissue pathologies and septa because certain pathologies and forms of septa might present contraindications to this procedure.
	Acquire consent. Give the patient enough time to go over consent forms and the opportunity to express any questions or concerns, and then obtain a signature. More than one consent form may be needed (eg, one consent form for the implant placement in addition to the sinus augmentation and one consent form for the oral sedation, if utilized).
	Prescribe medication. Antibiotics, an anti-inflammatory drug, an analgesic, and an antibacterial mouthrinse are recommended.
	Administer anesthesia. Local anesthesia (infiltration or V2 block) and oral sedation are recommended; however, the clinician might elect to use intravenous sedation instead of oral.
	Make the incisions and reflect a full-thickness flap. The flap should be large enough to appreciate the alveolar bone's width, and the releasing oblique incisions should be superior enough and approximately 15 mm mesial and distal to the planned window borders.
	Create the bony window. The lateral wall is scored with a diamond round bur to outline the window, which should be around 15 mm in height and 20 mm in width, and then complete detachment of the bony window from the surrounding bone is verified. The inferior border of the window should be 2 to 3 mm above the floor of the sinus, and the mesial border of the window should be 2 to 3 mm distal to the mesial border of the sinus. A Piezotome can be used to perform this step, if available. To minimize the possibility of tearing the membrane during this step (or the subsequent step), the corners of the window should not be sharp (an oval-shaped window is preferred).

(cont)

	Elevate the sinus membrane. The sinus membrane is elevated completely off the floor of the sinus, the anterior wall, and the medial wall to the desired height. Just before elevating the sinus membrane, the bony window can be completely removed or advanced inward to serve as the new floor of the sinus.
	Place the bone graft material. The graft material consists of a collagen membrane or tape (eg, Oratape, Salvin) to line the ceiling of the elevated area, bone grafting mix (eg, a combination of allograft and xenograft), and another long-lasting, pliable resorbable membrane to cover the window such as Bio-Gide (Geistlich).
	Suture the flap closed. Tension-free primary closure is achieved using Vicryl (Ethicon) or Gore-Tex (W. L. Gore) suturing material.
	Take a final radiograph for the patient's records.
	Deliver the provisional restoration. It is important that the provisional prosthesis does not exert any pressure on the incision line or on the grafted site.
	Provide postoperative instructions. The patient should be given instructions regarding hygiene, diet, and medications (see Postoperative Instructions for Sinus Elevation Procedure Checklist, page 63).
	Explain the follow-up protocol. The patient must be seen the next day, in 2 weeks for suture removal, and then 5 to 7 months later when the grafted sinus is nearly ready for implant placement.

✓	3.1 Mini-implant or Narrow-Platform Implant Treatment Planning
	Perform a general health screening for possible existing risk factors or contraindications. (See the General Risk Factors Checklist, page 9.)
	Evaluate the CT scan for available bone (including accurate dimension measurements, evaluation of related anatomical landmarks, and possible pathologies). (See the CT Scan Evaluation Checklist, page 13.)
	Decide on the number of implants. If possible, the preferred numbers are 5 in the mandible and 6 in the maxilla.
	Plan the location of the implants. Note that 4 equally spaced implants are better than 5 poorly spaced implants.
	Determine the insertion protocol (flapless versus with a flap when alveoloplasty is required; this is dictated by the shape and width of the crestal bone).
	Maximize the implant diameter.
	Select the loading protocol (immediate loading versus a two-stage protocol/delayed hard reline pickup procedure) after the evaluation of bone density and force factors (see the Force Factors Checklist, page 50). When the initial stability is not optimal on all implants or when reflection of a flap is necessary, the delayed hard reline pickup procedure is recommended.
	Evaluate the existing dentures (for fit and occlusion) if new dentures will not be fabricated in conjunction with implant placement.
	Evaluate the denture-bearing soft tissue. Excess gingiva should be reduced to an optimal thickness of 2 to 3 mm by a laser or an electrosurgical unit before or during the mini-implant surgical placement stage.

(cont)

	Evaluate the available vertical restorative space using properly mounted diagnostic casts. Limited vertical restorative space in the occlusion might require alveoloplasty simultaneous to the surgical placement.
	Evaluate the patient's bite for any parafunctions (see the Functional Risk Factors Checklist, page 11). Patients with heavy bites or any parafunctions (bruxism, clenching, or tongue thrusting) should have a delayed prosthetic protocol/pickup procedure, not wear dentures at night, and have flat plane denture teeth.
	Prescribe a proper postoperative home and in-office oral hygiene regimen, which is vital for the longevity of the implant and the health of the peri-implant tissues.

✓	**Force Factors**
In addition to the treatment planning guidelines, the force factors below must be considered during the treatment planning stage:	
	Patient age. Implants are under higher stress in younger patients.
	Patient sex. Male patients usually have stronger chewing forces.
	Opposing dentition. An opposing removable prosthesis is a more favorable scenario for a mini-implant–supported prosthesis.
	Parafunctions. The existence of any parafunction (ie, bruxism, clenching, or tongue thrusting) negatively affects the prognosis of mini-implants.
	Location of the implants in the arch. Posterior implants are subject to higher chewing forces.
	Patient diet. It is very important that the patient follows a soft diet protocol during the first 3 months after implant placement.

✓	3.2 Mini-implant or Narrow-Platform Implant Placement: Flapless Protocol
	Acquire consent. Give the patient enough time to go over consent forms and the opportunity to express any questions or concerns, and then obtain a signature. More than one consent form may be required (eg, one consent form for the prosthetic procedures and one for the oral sedation, if utilized).
	Administer medication. Antibiotics, an anti-inflammatory drug, an analgesic, and an antibacterial mouthrinse are recommended.
	Administer anesthesia. Local anesthesia is usually adequate; however, intravenous or oral sedation may be used in addition.
	Place the surgical guide (if prepared before surgery). Laboratory-fabricated or computer-generated surgical guides can be used during implant placement, if desired.
	Perform the initial osteotomy. Always use copious irrigation with refrigerated sterile water or sterile saline.
	Take a radiograph of the osteotomy with a drill in the osteotomy site. This can help determine the angulation and positioning of osteotomies.
	Continue the osteotomy preparation. Once satisfied with the radiograph, continue the osteotomy based on the implant diameter and bone density type. In most cases, only one drill is needed to create the osteotomy site for mini-implants; however, when mini-implants more than 2 mm in diameter are placed in dense bone, a second drill is required to adequately widen the osteotomy. Insert the drill to a depth of only one-third to one-half the length of the implant.
	Irrigate the osteotomy site and use suction to remove any debris.

(cont)

	Place the implant to the desired level. Use the recommended tools (finger driver, thumb driver, and hand ratchet), do not over-tighten the implant, and do not touch the implant with gloves. A minimum initial stability of 35 Ncm torque should be obtained. During use of the placement tools, avoid lateral forces, which can affect the angulation of the implants. Implants can be placed in the osteotomy with or without irrigation.
	Take a final radiograph for the patient's records.
	Reline the denture. A decision should be made at this time whether an immediate loading protocol is indicated (in which case a pickup procedure would be performed immediately after placement) or if a delayed restoration phase is indicated as a result of less than optimal initial stability. For the restorative phase, see the related checklist; otherwise, at this time the denture is relieved (where the mini-implant heads extrude through the gingiva), and a soft reline material is used to reline the denture. For immediate loading and restoration, the initial torque should be between 35 and 45 Ncm on all implants. If initial torque is below this range, delayed restoration may be performed, or the implants may be removed to new locations with higher bone density.
	Provide postoperative instructions. The patient should be given instructions regarding hygiene, diet, and medications (see Postoperative Instructions for Implant Placement/GBR Checklist, page 59).

✓	3.3 Mini-implant or Narrow-Platform Implant Placement: Full-Thickness Flap Protocol
When the crestal ridge is too narrow, it is highly recommended to reflect a full-thickness flap to perform an alveoloplasty procedure to gain a wider crestal ridge. This enables the clinician to place wider-diameter implants more precisely in the center of the alveolar ridge.	
	Acquire consent. Give the patient enough time to go over consent forms and the opportunity to express any questions or concerns, and then obtain a signature. More than one consent form may be needed (eg, one consent form for the prosthetic procedures and one for the oral sedation, if utilized).
	Administer medication. Antibiotics, an anti-inflammatory drug, an analgesic, and an antibacterial mouthrinse are recommended.
	Administer anesthesia. Local anesthesia is usually adequate; however, intravenous or oral sedation may be used in addition.
	Reflect a full-thickness flap. The flap should be large enough to allow appreciation of the alveolar bone width, shape, and trajectory.
	Perform an alveoloplasty to flatten the crestal ridge. A minimum amount of bony ridge should be removed to achieve the goal of the alveoloplasty while avoiding the placement of short implants and staying at a safe distance from any anatomical landmarks (eg, the inferior alveolar nerve, the mental nerve and its anterior loop, and the sinus floor).
	Perform the initial osteotomy. Always use copious irrigation with refrigerated sterile water or sterile saline.
	Take a radiograph of the osteotomy with a drill in the osteotomy site. This can help determine the angulation and positioning of osteotomies.

(cont)

	Continue the osteotomy preparation. Once satisfied with the radiograph, continue the osteotomy based on the implant diameter and bone density type. In most cases, only one drill is needed to create the osteotomy site for mini-implants; however, when mini-implants more than 2.0 mm in diameter are placed in dense bone, a second drill is required to adequately widen the osteotomy. Insert the drill to a depth of only one-third to one-half the length of the implant.
	Irrigate the osteotomy site and use suction to remove any debris.
	Place the implant to the desired level. Use the recommended tools (finger driver, thumb driver, and hand ratchet), do not overtighten the implant, and do not touch the implant with gloves. A minimum initial stability of 35 Ncm torque should be obtained. During use of the placement tools, avoid lateral forces, which can affect the angulation of the implants. Implants can be placed with or without irrigation.
	Take a final radiograph for the patient's records.
	Reline the denture. When a flap is reflected, a hard reline pickup procedure is not recommended right away; instead, the clinician should perform a soft reline after adjusting the dentures to avoid any contact between the implant portion that is above the gingival level and the intaglio surface of the prosthesis. The hard reline pickup procedure can then be performed upon soft tissue healing in 1 to 2 months or after a period of 3 to 4 months if the initial stability was under 35 Ncm on any of the implants. For the restorative phase, see the related checklist.
	Provide postoperative instructions. The patient should be given instructions regarding hygiene, diet, and medications (see Postoperative Instructions for Implant Placement/GBR Checklist, page 59).
	Schedule follow-up appointments. Follow-up should occur the next day, then monthly until the hard reline pickup procedure visit, which is usually 1 to 4 months later as described above, and then twice a year.

3.4 Mini-implant and Narrow-Platform Implant Prosthetic Protocol

The prosthetic phase of restoring ball-type mini-implants or narrow-platform implants can occur immediately after placement if the initial stability and the bone density are satisfactory and flap elevation has not been performed. It should be delayed 2 to 4 months after implant placement if the initial stability was minimal, the bone density was less than optimal, or a flap elevation was necessary for placement.	
☐	Acquire consent. Give the patient enough time to go over consent forms and the opportunity to express any questions or concerns, and then obtain a signature.
☐	Transfer the implant locations to the prosthesis. Using indelible pencil, or Thompson sticks, mark the heads of the implants and transfer their location onto the intaglio surface of the prosthesis.
☐	Relieve the denture. Using an acrylic bur, create a trough or individual divots to allow for complete denture seating without any contact between the denture and the implants. Then place the O-ring caps and reseat the denture to verify complete seating without any contact between the denture and the caps.
☐	Perform a hard reline pickup.
The following steps should be performed after verification of adequate denture relief:	
☐	Apply a layer of petroleum jelly to the entire implant portion that is above the soft tissue level.
☐	Cut 1.5- to 2.0-mm pieces from the block-out shims.
☐	Place the shims and then the caps on the implants (ensure complete seating of the caps over the ball attachments of the implants).
☐	Fill the trough or divot areas of the denture generously to ensure that the denture will have tissue support between the metal housings and in the rest of the tissue-borne areas of the denture.
☐	Place the denture in the patient's mouth and ensure a firm bite in centric occlusion (excessive biting force should be avoided so as not to disturb the soft tissue architecture). Allow 5 to 10 minutes, according to the instructions for the hard reline material.

(cont)

	Remove and adjust the denture. Remove the denture and the shims from the denture or implant heads, and then trim and polish the tissue-borne surface of the denture.
	Perform a final check. Confirm that the fit and the occlusion of the denture have not been negatively affected by the pickup procedure, which might happen if the patient did not bite properly during the curing period for the hard reline material.
	Explain and schedule the follow-up protocol. If possible, the patient should not remove the dentures until the 48-hour follow-up visit. After that, the patient should be seen twice a year for routine cleanings. The O-rings should be replaced every 12 to 18 months as needed.
	Take a final radiograph for the patient's records.

✓	4.1 Postoperative Instructions for Implant Placement/GBR
	Take your prescribed medications (antibiotics, analgesics, anti-inflammatory medications, and chlorhexidine rinse) as directed.
	Avoid smoking.
	Avoid sucking liquid through a straw.
	Expect swelling, pain, and ecchymosis at the surgical site.
	Rest.
	During the 24-hour period following surgery, place light pressure and ice packs extraorally over the surgical site (15 minutes on/15 minutes off).
	In case of multiple implant placement, stay on a liquid diet for 2 days (Carnation Instant Breakfast, Meritene, and Ensure are recommended); then soft foods (the consistency of mashed potatoes or scrambled eggs) may be consumed following the second day and for at least 2 weeks (until the mucosal incision has closed completely).
	Do not wear a provisional prosthesis for 2 weeks. After 2 weeks, the provisional prosthesis can be worn, but you should not eat with it or wear it overnight.
	Do not lift or pull on the lip or cheek to look at the sutures.
	Do not brush or floss near the surgical site for a few days, and then brush and floss very lightly for 4 weeks before returning to routine brushing and flossing.
	In cases of immediate loading, avoid mastication on the implant crown for 6 to 8 weeks.
	Sutures should be removed in 2 weeks.
	Notify the office if your medications do not relieve discomfort or if you have questions.

✓	4.2 Postoperative Instructions for Socket Grafting
	Take your prescribed medications (antibiotics, analgesics, anti-flammatory medications, and chlorhexidine rinse) as directed.
	For the first 12 hours after surgery, place ice packs extraorally over the surgical site (15 minutes on/15 minutes off).
	A small amount of blood oozing from the surgical site is normal; in the event of such bleeding, bite down on sterile gauze for 30 to 45 minutes. However, if bleeding is excessive, contact the clinician's office immediately.
	Starting the second day after surgery, rinse with chlorhexidine or with warm salt water per the clinician's instructions.
	Follow a soft diet (foods the consistency of mashed potatoes or scrambled eggs) in the area of the surgery for 2 weeks.
	Avoid sucking on a straw, spitting, or smoking.
	Avoid brushing near the grafted site for 1 to 2 days.
	Relax as much as possible and avoid all strenuous activities for the first 24 hours following surgery.
	Contact the office if the you experience a fever of 101°F or higher, excessive bleeding, unusual pain, or reaction to the medications prescribed.
	Return for the postoperative follow-up and suture removal appointment.

(cont)

If a sinus communication occurred during surgery as a result of the close relationship between the roots of the maxillary teeth and the sinuses, these instructions should be followed:	
	Do not blow your nose.
	Do not sneeze through your nose but rather with your mouth open.
	Avoid swimming and strenuous exercise for at least 1 week.
	It is not uncommon to have a slight amount of bleeding from the nose for several days.
	If there is a persistent sinus communication, a second procedure occasionally may be required to close the communication.

✓	4.3 Postoperative Instructions for Block Grafting
	Take your prescribed medications (antibiotics, analgesics, anti-flammatory medications, and chlorhexidine rinse) as directed.
	Expect swelling, pain, and ecchymosis at the donor site (mandible).
	Relax as much as possible and avoid all strenuous activities for the first 24 hours following surgery.
	Do not pull on the lip or cheek in the region of the graft.
	Refrain from smoking because it will cause failure of the graft.
	Avoid chewing in the area of the graft until it has healed (a minimum of 14 days).
	Avoid sucking liquid through a straw.
	During the 24-hour period following surgery, place an ice pack with light pressure extraorally over the surgical site (15 minutes on/15 minutes off).
	Report bad taste and soreness or protruding screws immediately.
	Follow a liquid diet (Carnation Instant Breakfast, Meritene, and Ensure are recommended) for 2 days and then eat only soft foods (the consistency of mashed potatoes or scrambled eggs) for at least 2 weeks (until the mucosal incision has closed completely).
	Do not wear a prosthesis while eating or sleeping for 2 weeks.
	Avoid contact sports for 3 to 4 months.
	Contact the office if you experience a fever of 101°F or higher, excessive bleeding, unusual pain, or reaction to the medications prescribed.
	Avoid toothbrushing immediately after the surgery and the following day but resume the second day after surgery.

✓	4.4 Postoperative Instructions for Sinus Elevation Procedure
	Take your presrcibed medications (antibiotics, analgesics, anti-inflammatory medications, chlorhexidine rinse, nasal spray, and decongestant) as directed.
	Avoid smoking.
	Do not blow your nose for 2 weeks because this could create positive pressure, which could spread air though confluent soft tissue planes, creating soft tissue emphysema.
	Avoid sucking liquid through a straw because this creates negative intrasinus pressure.
	Try not to sneeze or cough; if it is unavoidable, keep the mouth open to decrease internal antral pressure.
	Some nasal bleeding (oozing of blood through the nose) may occur during the first day.
	Rest as much as possible for the first 3 to 7 days following surgery.
	During the 24-hour period following surgery, place light pressure and ice packs extraorally over the surgical site (15 minutes on/15 minutes off).
	Keep your head elevated. On the first night, your head should be elevated on two or more pillows. This will prevent airway obstruction and aspiration of blood and heavy saliva and will diminish edema.
	Maintain a liquid diet for 2 days (Carnation Instant Breakfast, Meritene, and Ensure are recommended); then soft foods (the consistency of mashed potatoes or scrambled eggs) may be consumed following the second day and for at least 2 weeks (until the mucosal incision has closed completely).
	Do not wear a prosthesis for 2 weeks.
	Do not lift or pull on the lip to look at the sutures.
	Return to the office for a postoperative checkup in 1 week.
	Notify the office if you feel granules in your nose, if your medications do not relieve discomfort, or if you have questions.

✓	4.5 Preoperative Sedation Instructions
	Plan to have someone nearby for the first 24 hours after surgery.
	Do not wear tight-fitting clothing such as tight T-shirts; instead, wear comfortable, loose, and preferably short-sleeved clothing. Bring along a lightweight jacket or sweater, and remove all jewelry from the neck and ears.
	Do not wear nail polish.
	Do not wear high heels or platform shoes because your reflexes may be slowed, making walking in them hazardous.
	Do not wear cosmetics, which can contaminate the surgical site.
	Know the names of any medications taken regularly and bring the medicines in their prescription containers on the day of your appointment.
	If you are diabetic, take half the prescribed dose of insulin in the morning of the dental appointment. (Patients with insulin-dependent diabetes will have early schedule priority.)
	Plan to spend a minimum of 2 hours in the office if you are being sedated.
	You may not leave alone. An adult must accompany you.
	You may not drive or operate a vehicle or heavy equipment.

✓	5.1 Basic Implant Placement Instrumentation Setup
	Implant retractor
	Minnesota retractor
	Seldin retractor
	Weider tongue retractor (for mandibular cases)
	Siegel round scalpel handle
	No. 15C blades
	Molt 9 periosteal elevator
	Rhodes chisel (used to clean the bone surface of any soft tissue after flap reflection)
	Adson serrated tissue forceps (nonlocking)
	Adson 1 × 2 tissue forceps (locking)
	Castroviejo caliper
	Iris curved cutting scissors
	Needle holder
	Periodontal probe
	Mouth mirror
	Disposable tissue punch (for implant placement using a flapless technique)
	Suture material (see the table at the end of this chapter for the recommended suturing material)

The instruments above are required in addition to the anesthesia instruments and supplies, implant surgical kit, surgical motor, implant contra-angle handpiece, disposable irrigation tubing, sterile saline, and disposable infection control supplies (eg, sterile gloves, masks, sterile nonwoven gauze, head caps, sterile bib, and sterile gowns).

✓	5.2 Immediate Implant Placement Instrumentation Setup
The instruments below are required in addition to the basic implant placement setup.	
	Periotome set
	Lucas currettes (small size)
	Luxators (straight, 3-, and 5-mm)
	Membrane placement instrument
	Smooth-tip membrane forceps
	Graft packer
	Graft material mixing cups
	Lindemann side-cutting drill
	Bone graft material
	Collagen membrane (required in some cases)

If available, the Piezotome (Acteon, Satelec) can be used instead of periotomes for atraumatic extraction.

✓	5.3 Postextraction Socket Grafting Instrumentation Setup
	Implant retractor
	Minnesota retractor
	Seldin retractor
	Weider tongue retractor (for mandibular cases)
	Periotome set
	Luxators (straight, 3-, and 5-mm)
	Teeth and root tip extraction forceps (might be needed in addition to the periotomes and the luxators)
	Lucas currettes (small size; for thorough debridment of the extraction socket after tooth removal)
	Sterile saline
	Membrane placement instrument
	Smooth-tip membrane forceps
	Graft material packer
	Graft material mixing cup
	Bone graft material (eg, allograft, xenograft, or alloplast)
	Collagen membrane (eg, collagen tape or collagen plug)
	Suture material (see Suturing Material recommendations, page 82)

The instruments above are required in addition to the anesthesia instruments and supplies and disposable infection control supplies (eg, sterile gloves, masks, sterile nonwoven gauze, head caps, sterile bib, and sterile gowns). If available, the Piezotome (Acteon, Satelec) can also be used to perform atraumatic extraction.

✓	5.4 GBR Instrumentation Setup
	Implant retractor
	Minnesota retractor
	Weider tongue retractor (for mandibular cases)
	Siegel round scalpel holder
	No. 15C blade
	Molt 9 periosteal elevator
	Rhodes chisel (used to clean the bone surface of any soft tissue after flap reflection)
	Straight surgical handpiece (1:1 ratio)
	Small round bur for straight surgical handpiece
	Periodontal probe
	Mouth mirror
	Prichard elevator
	Membrane placement instrument
	Smooth-tip membrane forceps
	Adson serrated tissue forceps (nonlocking)
	Adson 1 × 2 tissue forceps (locking)
	Bone graft material mixing cup

(cont)

	Iris curved cutting scissors
	Needle holder
	Tacking kit or screw fixation kit
	Suture material (see Suturing Material recommendations, page 82)

The instruments above are required in addition to the anesthesia instruments and supplies, surgical motor, disposable irrigation tubing, sterile saline, bone graft materials (eg, allograft, xenograft, alloplast, or rhBMP-2/ACS), membrane (eg, Bio-Gide [Geistlich], OraMem [Salvin], or titanium mesh), and disposable infection control supplies (eg, sterile gloves, masks, sterile nonwoven gauze, head caps, sterile bib, and sterile gowns). In addition, an implant surgical kit and contra-angle handpiece are needed if implants are to be placed simultaneously.

✓	5.5 Crestal Sinus Elevation Instrumentation Setup
	Implant retractor
	Minnesota retractor
	Siegel round scalpel handle
	No. 15C blade
	Disposable tissue punch (for implant placement using flapless technique)
	Molt 9 periosteal elevator
	Rhodes chisel (used to clean the bone surface of any soft tissue after flap reflection)
	Periodontal probe
	Mouth mirror
	Sinus osteotome kit with stoppers (Salvin)
	Mead mallet
	Membrane placement instrument
	Smooth-tip membrane forceps
	Graft material mixing cup
	Bone graft material
	Collagen membrane
	Graft material packer

(cont)

	Adson serrated tissue forceps (nonlocking)
	Adson 1 × 2 tissue forceps (locking)
	Iris curved cutting scissors
	Needle holder
	Sinuscope equipment (if sinuscope-controlled crestal sinus elevation technique is desired)
	Suture material (see Suturing Material recommendations, page 82)

The instruments above are required in addition to the anesthesia instruments and supplies, implant surgical kit, surgical motor, implant contra-angle handpiece, disposable irrigation tubing, sterile saline, and disposable infection control supplies (eg, sterile gloves, masks, sterile nonwoven gauze, head caps, sterile bib, and sterile gowns).

✓	5.6 Alveolar Ridge Expansion by Split-Ridge Technique Instrumentation Setup
	Implant retractor
	Minnesota retractor
	Siegel round scalpel handle
	No. 15C blade
	Molt 9 periosteal elevator
	Rhodes chisel (used to clean the bone surface of any soft tissue after flap reflection)
	Periodontal probe
	Mouth mirror
	Straight surgical handpiece (1:1 ratio)
	Round or oval alveoloplasty bur
	45-degree high-speed rear-exhaust surgical handpiece
	700 XXL tapered carbide surgical bur for high-speed surgical handpiece
	Ridge splitting/expansion chisel set (Salvin)
	Mead mallet
	Membrane placement instrument
	Smooth-tip membrane forceps
	Graft material mixing cup

(cont)

	Bone graft material
	Collagen membrane
	Graft material packer
	Adson serrated tissue forceps (nonlocking)
	Adson 1 × 2 tissue forceps (locking)
	Iris curved cutting scissors
	Needle holder
	Blunt-end dissection scissors (needed if muscle release is desired for extra flap tension release)
	Suture material (see Suturing Material recommendations, page 82)

The instruments above are required in addition to the anesthesia instruments and supplies, implant surgical kit, surgical motor, implant contra-angle handpiece, disposable irrigation tubing, sterile saline, and disposable infection control supplies (eg, sterile gloves, masks, sterile nonwoven gauze, head caps, sterile bib, and sterile gowns). Note that the use of a Piezotome (Acteon, Satelec) would eliminate the need for the high-speed surgical handpiece and the 700 XXL bur.

✓	5.7 Lateral Window Sinus Elevation Instrumentation Setup
	Implant retractor
	Minnesota retractor
	Dog bone retractor
	Molt mouth gag
	Siegel round scalpel handle
	No. 15C blade
	Molt 9 periosteal elevator
	Rhodes chisel (used to clean the bone surface of any soft tissue after flap reflection)
	Straight surgical handpiece (1:1 ratio)
	Round diamond bur for straight handpiece (no. 8 or no. 10)
	Sinus membrane elevation instrument set
	Graft material packer
	Graft material delivery syringe
	Kerrison rongeur 4-mm bite (Salvin) (needed when enlargement of the initial bony window is desired)
	Periodontal probe
	Mouth mirror
	Prichard elevator

(cont)

	Membrane placement instrument
	Smooth-tip membrane forceps
	Adson serrated tissue forceps (nonlocking)
	Adson 1 × 2 tissue forceps (locking)
	Bone graft material mixing cup
	Iris curved cutting scissors
	Needle holder
	Tacking kit
	Bone graft material (eg, allograft, xenograft, rhBMP-2/ACS, or a combination of two or more)
	Collagen membrane (eg, OraMem [Salvin] or Bio-Gide [Geistlich])
	Suture material (see Suturing Material recommendations, page 82)

The instruments above are required in addition to the anesthesia instruments and supplies, surgical motor, disposable irrigation tubing, sterile saline, and disposable infection control supplies (eg, sterile gloves, masks, sterile nonwoven gauze, head caps, sterile bib, and sterile gowns). If the addition of autogenous bone to the graft mix is desired, see the Intraoral Bone Harvesting Instruments and Devices Checklist, page 81. Note that the use of a Piezotome (Acteon, Satelec) would eliminate the need for the surgical handpiece.

✓	5.8 Grafting Using Allograft Block Instrumentation Setup
	Implant retractor
	Minnesota retractor
	Weider tongue retractor (for mandibular cases)
	Siegel round scalpel handle
	No. 15C blade
	Molt 9 periosteal elevator
	Rhodes chisel (used to clean the bone surface of any soft tissue after flap reflection)
	Straight surgical handpiece (1:1 ratio)
	Large round diamond bur for straight handpiece (no. 10) for recipient site preparation
	Straight fissure bur (for the creation of bleeding points)
	Periodontal probe
	Mouth mirror
	Prichard elevator
	Membrane placement instrument
	Smooth-tip membrane forceps
	Adson serrated tissue forceps (nonlocking)
	Adson 1 × 2 tissue forceps (locking)

(cont)

	Bone graft material mixing cup
	Iris curved cutting scissors
	Needle holder
	Block screw fixation kit
	Bone graft material (eg, allograft, xenograft, or a combination of the two)
	Collagen membrane (eg, Bio-Gide [Geistlich])
	Suture material (see Suturing Material recommendations, page 82)

The instruments above are required in addition to the anesthesia instruments and supplies, surgical motor, disposable irrigation tubing, sterile saline, and disposable infection control supplies (eg, sterile gloves, masks, sterile nonwoven gauze, head caps, sterile bib, and sterile gowns). If the addition of autogenous bone around the block is desired, see the Intraoral Bone Harvesting Instruments and Devices Checklist, page 81.

✓	5.9 Materials, Devices, and Instrumentation for Bleeding and Airway Control
It is highly recommended that all implant practices have the items below available for possible surgery-related emergencies (in addition to the emergency medical kit, emergency oxygen cylinder, vital signs monitor, and defibrillator). The entire staff must be trained in the use of the devices and instruments below in addition to CPR.	
	Bone wax (for bone surface bleeding)
	Collagen tape or plug (for excessive osteotomy and socket bleeding)
	Hemostatic gauze (for soft tissue bleeding)
	Straight and curved Kelly hemostat (for soft tissue bleeding)
	Gore-Tex (W. L. Gore) suture material (CV-4 and CV-5) for ligating exposed or buried bleeders
	Electrosurgical unit with proper coagulation tips (for soft and hard tissue bleeding control)
	Single-use emergency suction (for excessive bleeding)
	Guedel airways (for airway control)
	Laryngeal mask airways (for airway control)
	Emergency cricothyrotomy kit (for airway control)
	Manual single-use resuscitator (for airway control)

✓	5.10 Intraoral Bone Harvesting Instruments and Devices
One or more of the instruments on this list can be added to any bone grafting instrumentation list if the use of autogenous bone is desired.	
	Rushkin rongeur with 5-mm bite (used to harvest bone from the tuberosity area)
	10-mm bone harvesting trephine drill (used to harvest bone from the chin)
	6-mm bone harvesting trephine drill (used to harvest bone from the anterior maxilla, the tuberosity, the ramus, or the chin)
	Bruns bone curette (used to harvest cancellous bone from the chin after the block harvest)
	MX-grafter (Maxilon) (single-use instrument for harvesting bone from the maxillary or mandibular bone surfaces)
	Bone mill (for crushing autogenous bone after harvesting)

5.11 Suturing Materials

Recommended suture material	Indication
Gore-Tex (W. L. Gore) PTFE suture material CV-4	Main suture material used by the author in surgical oral implantology
Gore-Tex (W. L. Gore) PTFE suture material CV-5	To replace CV-4 when the oral mucosa is thin
Vicryl 4-0 (Ethicon) (or P-3 reverse cutting needle)	To replace CV-4 when the oral mucosa is thin and a small needle size is needed because of limited access
Prolene 6-0 (Ethicon) (Polypropylene) blue monofilament (on P-3 reverse cutting needle)	In the esthetic zone when the oral mucosa is thin
Vicryl 7-0 (Ethicon) (on P-1 reverse cutting needle)	To suture the lip or the skin (eg, accidental cut to the lip or the skin during surgical procedures)
Silk (eg, 4-0 or 5-0 on C-6 reverse cutting needle)	As a temporary suture material (eg, tying the flap away from the surgical field temporarily while performing the procedure)
Chromic Gut 4-0 (on C-6 reverse cutting needle)	In soft tissue grafting procedures (eg, tying the connective tissue graft to the recipient site before suturing the flap)

PTFE, polytetrafluoroethylene.

✓	6.1 Nerve Injury Evaluation
	Document a detailed description of the patient's complaint (type and duration of altered sensation, severity of affected sensation, and the area involved), and then perform the following 4 steps within a few days of surgery.
	Refer the patient for a CT scan to determine if an implant is impinging on a nerve.
	If there is nerve impingement, remove or withdraw the implant(s) clear of the nerve.
	Prescribe 800 mg of ibuprofen three times daily for 3 weeks because the cause of the altered sensation could be postoperative edema or a sequela of soft tissue manipulation.
	Perform the related altered sensation tests (see page 86).
	Repeat the examination 1 month later. If there is no improvement, follow the next 2 steps; otherwise, follow-up appointments should be scheduled to document progress.
	Refer the patient to a microneurosurgeon within 4 months of the injury.
	Consult your malpractice insurance provider for guidance.

Symptoms of Nerve Injury

After nerve injury, patients will experience one or more of the following symptoms:

- Paresthesia: burning sensation, numbness, or prickling
- Hypoesthesia: reduced feeling
- Hyperesthesia: increased sensitivity
- Dysesthesia: painful sensation
- Anesthesia: complete loss of feeling in the teeth, surrounding skin, and mucosa

(cont)

Spontaneous return of normal sensation after nerve injury depends on both the severity of the injury and the nerve involved. Partial transection of the lingual nerve is less likely to result in spontaneous resolution of symptoms than is a similar injury involving the inferior alveolar nerve, which has a bony canal to contain and direct the regeneration fibers.

Techniques for Evaluation of Altered Sensations

When lingual nerve injury is suspected, the sensation of the tongue can be tested with the use of salt and sugar. The sensitivity of the lip and gingiva for suspected inferior alveolar nerve and mental nerve injuries can be done using a cotton swab to determine sensitivity, ice and a warmed mirror handle to determine if the patient feels cold and heat, and a soft brush to assess the patient's ability to determine the direction of movement on the lip and chin with the eyes closed.

	6.2 Bleeding Management
	Call 911 at the first sign of swelling (especially when it is in the floor of the mouth).
	Maintain hand pressure. The bleeding artery must be pressed against a bony structure (ie, the greater palatine artery against the hard palate). However, when there is bleeding in the floor of the mouth, using one hand, press with the thumb intraorally and with the index finger extraorally on the suspected perforation site (Fig 1).

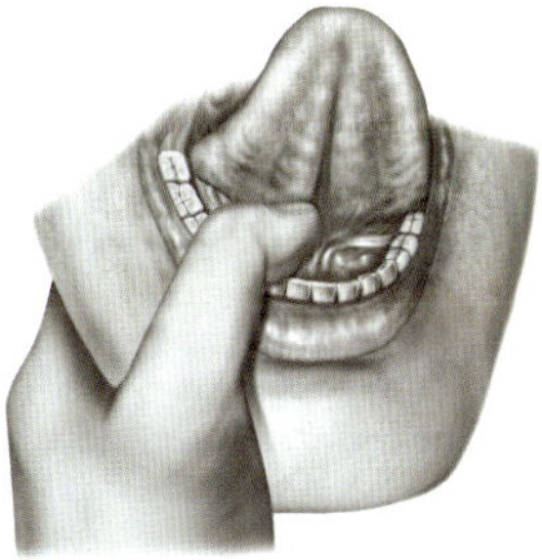

Fig 1

	Calmly explain to the patient the nature of the complication.
	Ligate the bleeding vessel. For buried bleeding vessels, the technique shown in Fig 2 can be used to attempt to ligate the vessel by applying pressure on the source of bleeding. Conversely, if the bleeding vessel can be identified and isolated, then its lumen can be closed by securing it with the tips of a small hemostat and placing a knot close to the lumen of the vessel.

(cont)

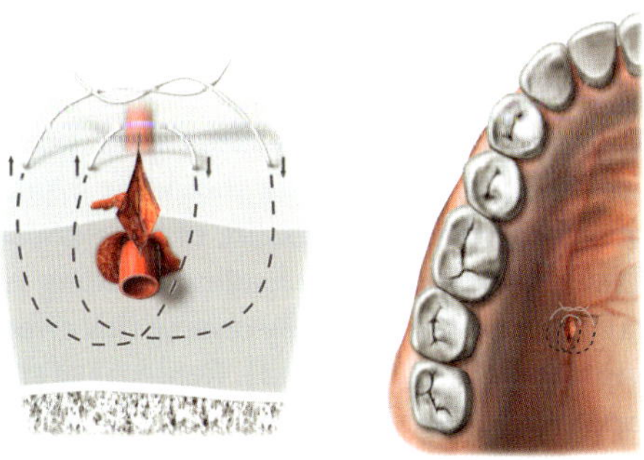

Fig 2

	Pull the tongue. Pulling the tongue forward (using Young forceps) against the hyoid bone will keep the airway open and reduce bleeding if the source of the bleeding is the lingual artery (Fig 3).

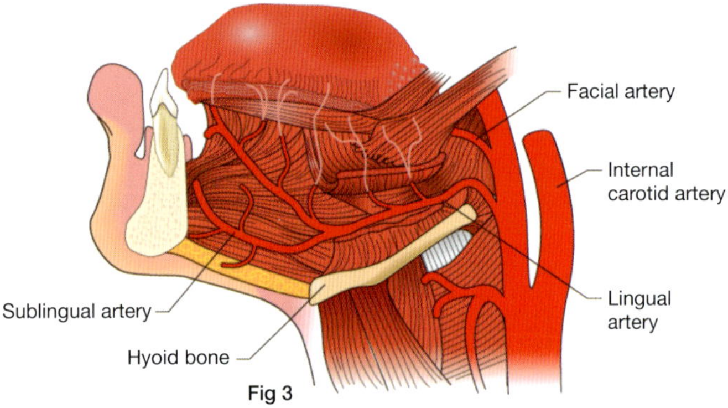

Fig 3

	Keep the airway open. If, despite application of all the techniques described above, a hematoma of large size develops in the floor of the mouth along with signs of respiratory distress, insertion of a flexible nasal airway should be performed (Guedel or laryngeal mask airway), or emergency tracheotomy or cricothyrotomy might be necessary (see the related checklist, page 89). The airway must be kept open until the paramedic service arrives.
	Transfer the patient to the hospital. Patient should be transferred to a nearby hospital for monitoring.
	Allow surgical intervention by a vascular surgeon. Once the bleeding has slowed, it can be stopped by surgical ties, electrocautery, or hemostasis after clot formation.

DO NOT

- Make any incisions to the floor of the mouth. Incisions in the floor of the mouth to relieve the hematoma should be avoided because the bleeding may stop when the pressure of the extravasated blood exceeds the vascular pressure of the feeding bleeding vessel. Therefore, hematoma drainage could potentially reverse this effect.
- Remove the implant (if already placed). Removal of the implant is not effective in stopping the bleeding.

6.3 Traditional Surgical Cricothyrotomy

✓	Required Equipment
	Scalpel with no. 15 blade
	Trousseau dilator (or small, curved hemostat)
	Tape
	Syringe
	Povidone iodine swab sticks
	Tracheostomy tube (or cuffed 6.0 endotracheal tube)
	Resuscitation bag

✓	Procedure
	Place the patient in a supine position, stabilize the neck region by placing a pillow or piece of cloth under the patient's shoulders, hyperextend the neck, and then, if povidone iodine/iodophor swab sticks are available, use them to disinfect the neck region.
	Stabilize the larynx with your nondominant hand by grasping the sides of the thyroid cartilage with your thumb and middle finger, and palpate the depression over the cricothyroid membrane using your index finger (the membrane is just inferior to the thyroid prominence and superior to the cricoid cartilage) (Fig 1).

(cont)

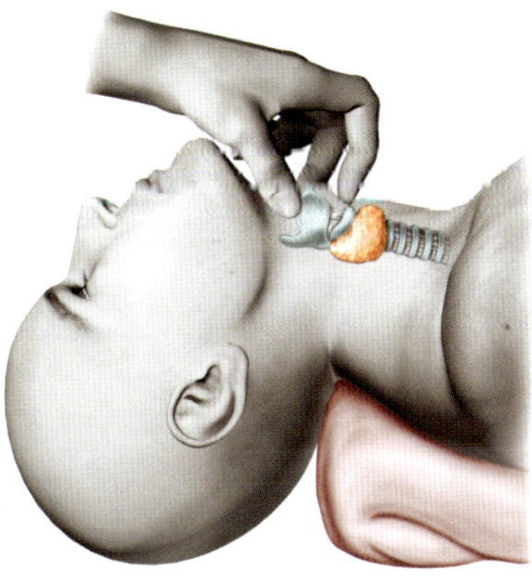

Fig 1

	Use the scalpel with no. 15 blade to make a 3-cm vertical incision through the skin and subcutaneous tissue overlying the cricothyroid membrane.
	Palpate the cricothyroid membrane using your index finger.
	Make a stabbing horizontal incision through the lower portion of the cricothyroid membrane (Fig 2).
	Place the Trousseau dilator into the trachea, then spread its blades open to dilate the opening in a vertical direction (do not insert the dilator too deep).
	Insert the airway into the trachea so that it is oriented parallel to the Trousseau dilator (while maintaining control of the Trousseau dilator), then rotate both together 90 degrees while advancing the tube further, and remove the Trousseau dilator.
	Insert the airway until the flange of the device rests against the patient's neck.
	Remove the obturator.
	Inflate the cuff with air.
	Secure the airway with tape.
	Begin to ventilate the patient using a resuscitation bag or ventilation circuit (Fig 3).

(cont)

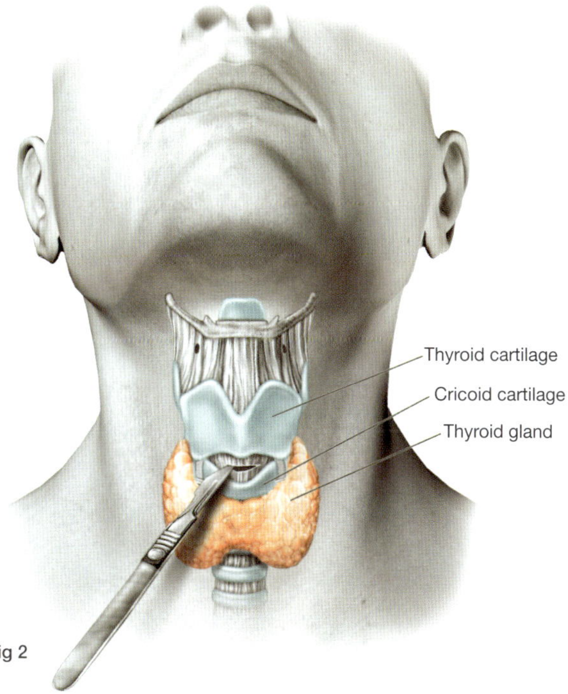

Fig 2

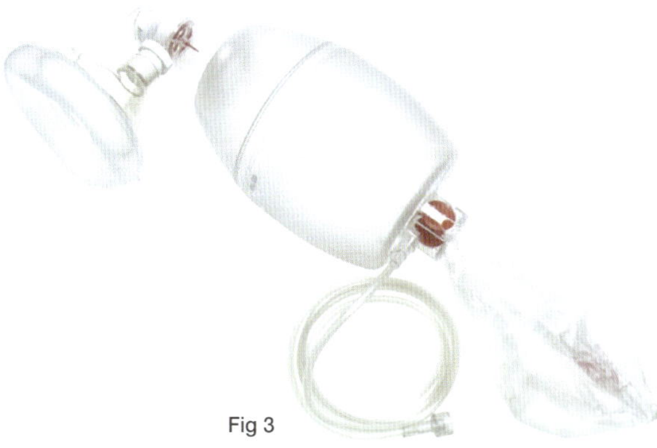

Fig 3